Ketogenic Bread

35 Low-Carb Keto Bread, Buns, Bagels, Muffins, Waffles, Pizza Crusts, Crackers & Breadsticks for Weight Loss and Healthy Living

By

Andrea J. Clark

Copyright © 2017 by Andrea J. Clark

All rights reserved. This book or any portion thereof may not be reproduced or used in any manner whatsoever without the express written permission of the publisher except for the use of brief quotations in a book review.

Disclaimer

This publication contains the opinions and ideas of its author. It is intended to provide helpful and informative material on the subjects addressed in the publication. It is sold with the understanding that the author and the publisher are not engaged in rendering medical, health, or any other kind of personal or professional services in the book. The reader should consult his or her medical, health or other competent professional before adopting any of the suggestions in this book.

The author and publisher are not responsible for the results that come from the application of the content within this book. This applies to risk, loss, personal or otherwise. This also applies to both direct and indirect application of the information contained in this publication.

Facebook: https://www.facebook.com/cleaneatingspirit

Instagram: https://www.instagram.com/cleaneatingspirit

Table of Contents

INTRODUCTION 1

CHAPTER ONE: OFTEN-USED KETOGENIC BREAD INGREDIENTS 6

CHAPTER TWO: KETOGENIC BREAD LOAVES 11
- CINNAMON BREAD 11
- COCONUT ROSEMARY BREAD 14
- CORN BREAD 16
- HERB BREAD 18
- JALAPEÑO BACON BREAD 20
- KETO PUMPKIN LOAF 22
- THANKSGIVING BREAD 25

CHAPTER THREE: KETOGENIC BUNS & BAGELS 28
- CAULIFLOWER BUNS 28
- KETO BUNS 31
- LOW-CARB EASY BAGELS 33
- MULTI-SEED BAGELS 36
- SESAME BUNS 39
- SUGAR-FREE BAGELS 42

CHAPTER FOUR: KETOGENIC MUFFINS, PANCAKES & WAFFLES 45
- ALMOND FLOUR WAFFLES 45
- CHEESE MUFFINS 47
- CREAM CHEESE PANCAKES 50
- GLUTEN-FREE LOW-CARB PANCAKES 52
- LEMON BLUEBERRY MUFFINS 54
- LOW-CARB CINNAMON WAFFLES 56
- LOW-CARB SOUR CREAM BLUEBERRY MUFFINS 59

CHAPTER FIVE: KETOGENIC PIZZA CRUST 61
- CAULIFLOWER CRUST 61

- EASY ALMOND FLOUR PIZZA CRUST 64
- LOW-CARB PIZZA CRUST 66
- KETO CAULIFLOWER CRUST 69
- PARMESAN AND ALMOND PIZZA CRUST 72

CHAPTER SIX: KETOGENIC CRACKERS 75
- CHEESY KETO CRACKERS 75
- GRAIN-FREE KETO CRACKERS 78
- KETO PESTO CRACKERS 81
- LOW-CARB FLAXSEED CRACKERS 84
- LOW-CARB SEA SALT CRACKERS 86

CHAPTER SEVEN: KETOGENIC BREADSTICKS 88
- CAULIFLOWER CHEESE BREADSTICKS 88
- CHEESY GARLIC BREADSTICKS 91
- KETO BREADSTICKS 94
- PIZZA BREADSTICKS 97
- SESAME LOW-CARB BREADSTICKS 100

CONCLUSION 103
AUTHOR'S NOTE 105

Introduction

The Ketogenic Diet (keto) is a low-carbohydrate diet and converts the human body into a fat-burning machine. The diet is akin to other low-carb diets like LCHF (low-carb, high-fat) and the Atkins Diet. These diets – more or less accidentally – end up being keto.

The keto diet can improve your health via a metabolic switch in the main cellular fuel source to which the brain and body are adapted. When the metabolism shifts from depending on carb-based fuels (glucose from sugar and starch) to fat-based fuels and ketones (which are fat metabolism products), positive changes in your cells' health occur. This means better overall health.

Ketogenesis – a metabolic process – and ketosis – a body state – are responsible. Simply put, ketosis is a conventional metabolic pathway in which the brain and body cells use ketones to provide energy, instead of depending on carbohydrates and other conventional sugars.

Humans, in fact, developed an evolutionary capability to burn off ketones as an adaptation to long durations of food unavailability.

Moreover, being in nutritional ketosis is a body state that is beneficial.

Research is done on ketosis and its relationship to disease. Ketone bodies can benefit the human body, and elevating the blood levels with ketone bodies is effective to treat various diseases as they improve mitochondrial health and cellular energy pathways' function.

Aside from promoting overall health, the keto diet is being looked into to treat medical conditions like epilepsy, diabetes, Alzheimer's disease, autism, cancer, and other conditions. Much of the treatments' success is rooted in cellular effects.

A keto diet plan entails tracking the amount of carbs in the food eaten and reducing carb intake to around 20 to 60 grams daily. For certain people, less than 100 grams of daily carbs may work, but such carb level intake may be too high for most people to achieve ketosis.

When there is no calorie restriction, a keto diet's nutrient intake normally works out to around 70 to 75% fat calories, 20 to 25% protein calories, and around 5 to 10% carbohydrate calories.

The key to proper implementation of a keto diet is to keep in mind that you are exchanging carb-containing food with a moderate protein consumption and higher fat intake.

Benefits of the Ketogenic Diet

Choosing a keto diet offers valuable health benefits. Research indicates that being in a nutritional ketosis state leads to vital improvements in weight loss and blood glucose control, among others.

Some other common benefits of the keto diet include:

- Improvements in insulin sensitivity,
- Reduced medication dependence,
- Lower blood pressure,
- Improved cholesterol levels,
- Stronger mental performance,
- Reducing food cravings,
- Reducing sugary food preference,
- Helping you feel full longer, and
- Reduce yeast infections and thrush that can lead to candida.

What to Eat on the Keto Diet

Regarding certain food to include on a low-carb or keto diet, and those to avoid or limit, below are food items that you may consider for your keto diet grocery list.

To Eat

- Eat various **vegetables**, especially: mushrooms, leafy greens carrots, tomatoes, cabbage, broccoli, spinach,

Brussels sprouts, sea vegetables, kale, peppers, and many others.

- **Healthy fats**, which are also no-carb or low-carb, include: coconut oil, olive oil, palm oil, grass-fed butter, seeds, and nuts.

- Healthy food choices that are rich in **protein** but no-carb or low-carb include: pasture-raised poultry, grass-fed beef, cage-free eggs, wild-caught fish, bone broth protein, raw daily products like goat cheese (raw), and organ meats.

- If you have to add **carbohydrates** to your meals, choose those that are unprocessed and complex. You may consume sweet potatoes; ancient or sprouted grains like quinoa, oats, amaranth, buckwheat, and brown rice; legumes and beans; whole fruits; and, in small amounts, natural or artificial sweeteners like raw honey, stevia, or Splenda.

To Avoid

- Avoid ultra-processed and **processed food** high in calories. These processed food are also lacking in terms of nutrients. Avoid food items like: those made with wheat flour or white flour products, conventional dairy, added table sugar, bread and processed grains like pasta, sweetened snacks like cakes and cookies, sweetened drinks, most box cereals, and ice cream.

What You Will Learn from this Book

While this book touches on the basics of what the Ketogenic diet is, it focuses more on bread-based recipes that you can use while you are on the keto diet. We do need our everyday staples, right? We have been so used to eating a carbohydrate-based staple to accompany our protein dishes, and we may be at a loss as we start to transition to the keto diet. It can be difficult for us to do away with our staple food.

The recipes that follow are keto variations of your favorite staples. The difference is that they use ingredients that are keto-friendly. Instead of conventional wheat flour, the recipes use almond flour, coconut flour, or even cauliflower. Moreover, the end products are just as tasteful as their wheat-based counterparts – only more nutritious.

Thus, you do not have to be glum while you are on the keto diet. You can still eat your favorite staples like breads, muffins, pancakes, waffles, pizzas, crackers, bagels, buns, and breadsticks.

Not only will you enjoy eating the keto food based on the recipes that follow, you can – in time – derive the health benefits of sticking to the keto diet. You will lose a healthy amount of unwanted weight, you gain mental clarity, you are disease-free, and you achieve overall health.

Chapter One: Often-Used Ketogenic Bread Ingredients

You do not have to fight carbohydrates entirely as you switch to the keto diet for overall health. You only need to make smart substitutions on ingredients that are thought of as not beneficial to your health in the long term.

Navigating your way around the kitchen to make nutritious and delicious keto-friendly food is the end goal here. From cooking to baking, you need the appropriate ingredients to push the flavors to the next level and help you love what you prepare and eat.

Cooking ketogenic-friendly food can be a challenge already when it comes to knowing the right substitutions for traditional ingredients. Below are some often-used ketogenic-friendly ingredients that you can use as you prepare the following keto-friendly breads.

Flour

All-purpose flour is a no-no on the ketogenic diet, so you need substitutes to bake your breads and muffins. An alternative to regular flour is almond flour, which has more fat, lesser carbohydrates, and has only a bit of protein. While almond flour takes getting used to, this will eventually become a staple in keto-based baked goods.

Coconut flour can be another staple in the ketogenic kitchen. Coconut flour is more absorbent than almond flour. The flour can also be used as a thickener, and is a versatile kitchen staple. With a much lower omega-6 count, a lot of people bank on the health benefits of coconut.

While not exactly called a flour, Psyllium husk is a staple in most of this book's recipes. It is absorbent and contributes to that whole-wheat flavor. It also provides a texture that is akin to whole grain flour.

Thus, when you are making bread, tortillas, or muffins, Psyllium can give you that extra flavor and texture. Psyllium husk's taste provides a baked wheat effect and gives wheat flour's realistic texture.

Sweetener: Powder and Liquid Sugar Substitute

Conventional white sugar is an absolute no-no in the keto diet. However, Mother Nature and modern chemistry have provided you the right sweeteners to help you stick to your regimen. One such sweetener is stevia. From lowering diabetics' blood sugar levels to lowering blood pressure and cholesterol, stevia should be a staple in the keto kitchen. Moreover, it has a zero glycemic index and has proven health benefits.

Another sugar substitute is erythritol. While nutrition labels say erythritol has carbohydrates, the body lacks the enzymes to break down the sweetness's source. About 90% of the sweetener goes through the digestive system and is accordingly excreted. Swerve is a sweeter made from a combination of erythritol and oligosaccharides (from chicory root). This aids the cooling sensation sometimes tasted when using erythritol alone in baking.

Chocolate, Coconut Products

Dark chocolate bars are preferable in the ketogenic diet. With dark chocolate, look for a product that has a higher cocoa percentage – like 86%. You can also use cocoa powder, but go for the unsweetened and dark types where you can control the sweetness's amount. Cocoa powder is excellent for baked or non-baked goods like puddings, cookies, and cakes, and where you desire an overall chocolate taste.

A coconut-based product like coconut oil can substitute the standard oils used in baked breads and other baked products. Coconut oil can reduce cravings for hunger and can keep you fuller for longer.

Fruits

You can use fruit in the keto diet, but you have to choose the fruits that are relatively lower in carbohydrates. Some low-carb fruit options include peaches, rhubarb, starfruit, casaba melon, watermelon, and grapefruit.

At least in the beginning of your keto diet regimen, it is best to limit or avoid berries. Who would not want berries? Thankfully, there are fruit extracts in a variety of flavors. Do you want to enjoy blueberry muffins? You can use a blueberry extract for that.

Nuts

Nuts and seeds are go-to foods in the ketogenic diet, and such food items present their own set of benefits to baking and the health. Almonds are crunchy, delicious, and add texture to almost any bread. You can also make your own nut butter with almonds.

Macadamia nuts are high in fat. You can bake them in brownies or sprinkle them in cream cheese. The fat content in walnuts is almost as high as in macadamias. Walnuts, however, are softer and more decadent, and are great for sprinkling on cream-based toppings.

Pecans, which almost have a butter flavor, go well with maple. Thus, if you are cooking waffles, pancakes, cupcakes, or muffins, pecans are the right fit. While not a nut, the nutrient-rich chia seeds are high in fat and low on carbs. They are also packed with magnesium, calcium, and phosphorus. Chia seeds are an excellent addition to cookies, brownies, and puddings.

Chapter Two: Ketogenic Bread Loaves

CINNAMON BREAD

You may be hesitant to try out coconut flour for the first time, but you may find out that using it is flavorful. It is interesting to know that coconut flour alone is cheaper than using almond flour. Plus, the cinnamon adds a delightful aroma that reminds you of home.

Serves: 10

Prep Time: 5 minutes

Cook Time: 25 minutes

Ingredients:

- ½ cup coconut flour
- ½ teaspoon baking powder
- ½ teaspoon baking soda
- 1 teaspoon cinnamon
- 1 teaspoon vinegar
- 3 eggs, pastured

- 1/8 teaspoon stevia (organic) or choice sweetener, to taste
- 3 tablespoons butter, salted
- 1/3 cup Greek yogurt or sour cream (For a dairy-free option, you can use coconut oil and coconut milk added with 1/8 teaspoon salt.)
- 2 tablespoons water

Directions:

1. Preheat the oven to 350°F (175°C). Use parchment paper to line a greased loaf pan. Combine the dry ingredients and whisk them together until blended.
2. Add the rest of the ingredients and combine them well. Taste for sweetness and adjust accordingly if needed. Allow the batter to stand and mix again.
3. If you are using a natural sweetener, add 2 tablespoons of coconut sugar to the batter.
4. Pour the batter into the prepared loaf pan. Bake for 25 to 30 minutes, or until a toothpick inserted in the middle comes out clean.
5. Remove from oven. Cool the bread on wire rack, and store it in the refrigerator before serving.
6. Slice and serve.

Nutrition Facts per Serving:

Total Carbs: 1.68 g

Dietary Fiber: .28 g

Net Carbs: 1.4 g

Total Fat: 7.44 g

Protein: 3.35 g

Calories: 90 kcal

COCONUT ROSEMARY BREAD

This coconut rosemary bread is a good accompaniment for paleo pates or soups. The bread's lighter texture, coupled with the aromatic rosemary flavor, is great to enjoy during the summers.

Serves: 10

Prep Time: 20 minutes

Cook Time: 45 minutes

Ingredients:

- 4 eggs
- ¼ cup coconut milk
- ¼ cup olive oil
- 1 teaspoon sea salt
- 1 teaspoon baking soda
- 1 teaspoon rosemary, freshly ground
- ¾ cup coconut flour
- 1/3 cup flaxseed meal

Directions:

1. Preheat the oven to 350°F (175°C).
2. In a large bowl, use a hand mixer to beat the olive oil, eggs, rosemary, and coconut milk. Mix until smooth.
3. Add the baking soda, sea salt, and flaxseed meal. Mix well.
4. Add the coconut flour. Mix well. The mixture should be dry at this point.
5. Use a spatula to scrape off the dough, and pour it into an oven-proof dish. Use your hands to form the dough into a bread shape. You may also scoop the dough into a baking tin, and use your spatula to spread out the dough.
6. Bake for 45 minutes, or until a toothpick that you inserted comes out clean.
7. Remove from oven. Cool and serve.

Nutrition Facts per Serving:

Total Carbs: 3.02 g

Dietary Fiber: 1.85 g

Net Carbs: 1.17 g

Total Fat: 13.06 g

Protein: 4.87 g

Calories: 146.40 kcal

CORN BREAD

This corn bread's savory taste makes it perfect for stews and soups. To bulk up the loaf, leave the eggs in room temperature. However, it is vital not to overheat the oil, or the eggs may be inadvertently cooked.

Serves: 10

Prep Time: 35 minutes

Cook Time: 40 minutes

Ingredients:

- 1 cup water
- 4 eggs
- ½ cup coconut flour
- 2 tablespoons apple cider vinegar
- ¼ cup and 1 teaspoon coconut oil, melted
- ½ teaspoon garlic powder
- ½ teaspoon baking soda
- ¼ teaspoon coarse sea salt

Directions:

1. Place the eggs in room temperature. One way is to crack them in a blender and allow them to sit for about 20 minutes.
2. Add the water, apple cider vinegar, and ¼ cup melted coconut oil. Make sure the oil is not too hot. Blend the ingredients for 30 seconds on low.
3. Mix in the garlic powder, coconut flour, baking soda, and salt. Blend for one minute.
4. Use 1 teaspoon coconut oil to grease a baking tin. You can use two small loaf pans.
5. Pour the batter into the baking tin or two small tins. Bake for 40 to 45 minutes at 350°F (175°C), or until an inserted toothpick comes out clean.
6. To achieve a golden look, an option is to rub 1 teaspoon coconut oil on top of the loaf or loaves. Do this one minute before you remove the bread from the oven. Broil on low until you achieve the desired color.
7. Remove from oven and cool. Serve and enjoy.

Nutrition Facts per Serving:

Total Carbs: 1.31 g

Dietary Fiber: .15 g

Net Carbs: 1.16 g

Total Fat: 9.33 g

Protein: 3.7 g

Calories: 103 kcal

HERB BREAD

With this bread, you can use various flavors and herbs. If you have no fresh herbs around, you can use dried herbs. Cut back the amounts as dried herbs tend to have a stronger flavor.

Serves: 10

Prep Time: 10 minutes

Cook Time: 30 minutes

Ingredients:

- 1 ½ cups almond flour, blanched
- 2 tablespoons coconut flour
- 2 tablespoons chopped herbs of choice (thyme and rosemary are acceptable)
- 2 tablespoons flaxseed meal
- 1 ½ teaspoons baking soda
- ¼ teaspoon sea salt
- 5 eggs
- 1 tablespoon apple cider vinegar
- ¼ cup melted coconut oil

Directions:

1. Preheat oven to 350°F (175°C), and grease a loaf pan. Set the pan aside.
2. In a food processor, place the almond flour, flax, coconut flour, salt, herbs, and baking soda. Pulse together and combine well. Pulse in the oil, eggs, and vinegar.
3. Pour the batter into the prepared pan. Bake for 25 to 30 minutes or until the bread looks golden and a toothpick inserted in the pan's center comes out clean.
4. If the top of the bread is getting too brown in under 30 minutes, put a piece of aluminum foil on top. This prevents the top from burning.
5. After baking, remove from oven. Cool before serving. You may top each serving with grass-fed butter, if desired.
6. If you do not have fresh herbs, use dried herbs but with lesser quantity. You can use ½ to 1 teaspoon each for your chosen dried herb. Aside from thyme and rosemary, you can use dried oregano or pizza seasoning.

Nutrition Facts per Serving:

Total Carbs: 5.30 g

Dietary Fiber: 2.75 g

Net Carbs: 2.55 g

Total Fat: 22.57 g

Protein: 9.54 g

Calories: 252 kcal

JALAPEÑO BACON BREAD

If you are serving a Mexican-inspired spread, this bread can be an additional delight. With the bacon, you can also serve it for breakfast or you can serve it as a side dish for chili. If you have leftovers or you do not plan to eat it immediately, store it in the refrigerator because of the number of eggs used.

Serves: 10

Prep Time: 20 minutes

Cook Time: 50 minutes

Ingredients:

- 3 pieces jalapeños, large
- 4 ounces bacon (about 4 thick slices)
- 6 eggs, large
- ½ cup melted ghee
- ½ cup coconut flour
- ¼ teaspoon baking soda
- ½ teaspoon sea salt
- ¼ cup water
- 1 tablespoon ghee, to grease baking pan

Directions:

1. Preheat oven to 400°F (205°C). Meanwhile, slice the jalapeños and arrange on a baking dish with the bacon slices. Once the oven is preheated, roast the bacon and the peppers for 10 minutes. Midway, flip the jalapeño and bacon slices.
2. Let the bacon and peppers slightly cool. Deseed the jalapeños. Put them in the food processor, and thoroughly pulse.
3. In a large bowl, mix together water, ghee, and eggs. Sift in the sea salt, coconut flour, and baking soda.
4. Into the batter, fold in the jalapeño-bacon mixture.
5. Grease a baking dish with one tablespoon of ghee. Pour in the batter. Bake at 375°F (190°C) for 40 to 45 minutes, or until an inserted toothpick comes out clean.
6. Cool for 10 to 15 minutes. Slice the bread and serve.

Nutrition Facts per Serving:

Total Carbs: 2.43 g

Dietary Fiber: .33 g

Net Carbs: 2.1 g

Total Fat: 20.65 g

Protein: 7.27 g

Calories: 223.1 kcal

KETO PUMPKIN LOAF

This dense bread is extremely satisfying and is great at the breakfast table. A slice or two of this delicious keto-friendly bread can set you up the entire morning.

Serves: 10

Prep Time: 15 minutes

Cook Time: 1 hour 15 minutes

Ingredients:

- 1 ½ cups almond flour
- ½ cup pumpkin puree
- 3 egg whites, derived from three large eggs
- ¼ cup Psyllium Husk powder
- ½ cup coconut milk (from carton)
- ¼ cup Swerve sweetener
- 1 ½ teaspoons pumpkin spice
- 2 teaspoons baking powder
- ½ teaspoon kosher salt

Pumpkin Spice Ingredients:

- 1 tablespoon ginger, ground
- 2 tablespoons cinnamon, ground
- ½ teaspoon allspice
- ½ teaspoon nutmeg, ground
- ¼ teaspoon cardamom
- ½ teaspoon cloves, ground

Directions:

1. To make the pumpkin spice, ready your spices and a small bowl. Mix all the spices in the bowl. Mix the spices together until you achieve a uniform color. Store in a spice container, and use as needed.
2. To make the bread, measure the dry ingredients out in a sifter. Sift the dry ingredients in a large bowl, and preheat the oven to 350°F (175°C).
3. Fill a baking dish (9" x 9") with one cup of water and place it on the oven's bottom rack.
4. Add in the coconut milk and pumpkin puree into the bowl, and mix well.
5. In another bowl, whip the egg whites. Add cream of tartar, if needed. Into the dough, fold in 1/3 of the egg whites. Do this aggressively to absorb moisture. Add the remaining egg whites and fold in gently.
6. Grease a bread loaf pan with coconut oil or butter, and then pour the dough into the pan.

7. Bake the bread for 1 hour and 15 minutes. If you desire, you can add pistachios on top, although the bread alone tastes good without them.

8. Remove the loaf and allow it to cool. Slice the bread and serve.

<u>Nutrition Facts per Serving:</u>

Total Carbs: 8.1 g

Dietary Fiber: 5 g

Net Carbs: 3.1 g

Total Fat: 8.7 g

Protein: 4.5 g

Calories: 119.6 kcal

THANKSGIVING BREAD

You can serve this during Thanksgiving in place of muffins. With the flavors of rosemary and sage, the taste of bacon, and a whiff of poultry, you can serve this bread with your turkey.

Serves: 10

Prep Time: 20 minutes

Cook Time: 35 minutes

Ingredients:

- 1 chopped onion
- 1 tablespoon ghee (organic) or fat of choice
- ½ cup walnuts
- 2 stalks chopped celery
- ½ cup coconut flour
- 1 ½ cups almond flour
- ¼ teaspoons sea salt, fine
- 1 teaspoon baking soda
- 1 tablespoon chopped rosemary, fresh
- Pinch of nutmeg, freshly grated

- 10 finely-chopped sage leaves
- ½ cup chicken broth
- 4 eggs
- 2 to 3 bacon strips, fried and crumbled (If you will not use bacon, add a bit more salt to your bread batter.)

Directions:

1. Preheat the oven to 350°F (175°C). Over medium heat, melt the ghee (or your choice shortening) in a pan.
2. Add the celery and onion to the ghee and sauté for around 5 minutes. Add the walnuts. Sauté for a couple more minutes. Set aside the mixture.
3. Combine the coconut flour, almond flour, salt, baking soda, rosemary, sage, and nutmeg in a large bowl. Mix the ingredients well.
4. Into the large bowl, add in the sautéed onion mixture. Add the chicken broth and eggs. Mix to combine well.
5. Fold in the cooked bacon bits into the bread batter.
6. Spread the batter into a standard loaf pan. Bake for about 35 minutes, or until an inserted toothpick in the center comes out clean.
7. Remove from oven and cool. Serve and enjoy.

Nutrition Facts per Serving:

Total Carbs: 4.33 g

Dietary Fiber: .91 g

Net Carbs: 3.42 g

Total Fat: 8.13 g

Protein: 4.84 g

Calories: 107.5 kcal

Chapter Three: Ketogenic Buns & Bagels

CAULIFLOWER BUNS

Who would have thought you can make ketogenic buns using cauliflower? The light and fluffy buns may taste like the vegetable, but the garlic powder adds a whole new zing to it. The nutritional yeast adds a cheese-like flavor.

Serves: 12

Prep Time: 20 minutes

Cook Time: 30 minutes

Ingredients:

- 1 cauliflower, large (1,200 g)
- ¼ cup nutritional yeast
- ¼ cup almond meal
- ½ teaspoon garlic powder
- 1 ½ teaspoon sea salt, fine
- 2 large eggs, organic

- 1 tablespoon Psyllium husk (an option, as it can make the buns drier)
- 1 tablespoon onion (dried) or sesame seeds

Directions:

1. Wash the cauliflower and chop it into chunks. Put in a food processor and process until fine. Do this in batches as the cauliflower cannot process well if the food processor is overly full.

2. Place the processed cauliflower into a large mixing bowl. Add the nutritional yeast, almond meal, garlic powder, salt, and psyllium husk (if you are using it). Stir thoroughly to combine.

3. Preheat the oven to 400°F (205°C).

4. In a separate bowl, whisk the eggs. Add them to the cauliflower mix, and stir until the mixture will hold together and is moist.

5. Use parchment paper to line a baking sheet. Use baseball-sized amounts of the 'dough,' and roughly squeeze them into a ball shape. Drop them from about 30 cm (1 foot) high on to the baking sheet.

6. Sprinkle the tops of the buns with sesame seed or dried onion.

7. Put in the oven and bake for 20 to 30 minutes, or until the edges of the buns are golden brown.

8. Serve. Enjoy the buns warm with grass-fed butter.

9. You may store leftovers in the refrigerator for 3 to 4 days.

Nutrition Facts per Serving:

Total Carbs: 5.17 g

Dietary Fiber: 1.89 g

Net Carbs: 3.28 g

Total Fat: 1.42 g

Protein: 3.40 g

Calories: 44.25 kcal

KETO BUNS

These buns can easily substitute English muffins for breakfast. They can be toasted, frozen, re-toasted. You can add a bit of grass-fed butter on top.

Serves: 6

Prep Time: 5 minutes

Cook Time: 26 minutes

Ingredients:

- 4 tablespoons melted lard (You can also use beef tallow or unsalted butter.)
- ½ teaspoon Himalayan salt
- 4 eggs
- 1 tablespoon rosemary
- 100 grams almond flour, blanched
- 1 tablespoon sesame seeds, black
- 1 tablespoon sesame seeds, white
- 1 teaspoon onion flakes

Directions:

1. Preheat the oven to 425°F (220°C).

2. Add the eggs and melted lard inside a blender. Add the remaining ingredients to the liquid mixture. Pulse for 5 to 10 times until the batter is thoroughly combined.
3. Equally pour the batter into 6 jumbo silicon muffin molds. If you desire, sprinkle the remaining sesame seeds over each bun.
4. Place the buns in the oven, and bake for 26 minutes. Remove the buns from the oven, and cool completely before cutting.

Nutrition Facts per Serving:

Total Carbs: 3.99 g

Dietary Fiber: 2.1 g

Net Carbs: 1.89 g

Total Fat: 20.82 g

Protein: 8.45 g

Calories: 230 kcal

LOW-CARB EASY BAGELS

The almond & cashew butter used in this recipe has a strong flavor, and the coconut flour can soak up the bagels' moisture. The flour also prevents the bagels from becoming too chewy.

Serves: 8

Prep Time: 10 minutes

Cook Time: 25 minutes

Ingredients:

- 4 eggs (large), separated, organic or free-range
- 1 cup almond butter or almond & cashew butter (8.8 ounces/250 g)
- ¼ cup lukewarm water
- ¼ cup lukewarm coconut milk or cream
- ¼ cup sifted coconut flour
- 1 teaspoon baking soda
- 1 teaspoon sea salt
- 2 teaspoons cream of tartar

Directions:

1. It is important to use nut butter that is warm. Cold nut butter from the refrigerator would be a challenge to mix. If

necessary, warm up the butter slightly in a microwave oven or a water bath.

2. Preheat oven to 400°F (205°C). Separate the eggs, and place the yolks into the warmed nut butter. Add baking soda. Season with salt and add lukewarm water and lukewarm coconut cream or milk. Use an electric mixer to combine the ingredients well.

3. In another bowl, beat the egg whites. While beating, add cream of tartar until the whites form soft peaks.

4. Pour the coconut flour into the bowl with the sticky dough. Combine until thoroughly mixed. Add the egg whites and process until combined well.

5. Spoon the dough into a bagel or doughnut pan. Bake for 5 minutes at 400°F (205°C). Lower the temperature to 300°F (150°C), and bake for a further 15 to 20 minutes.

6. Take the cooked bagels away from the oven to cool down.

7. Cut along the bagel's width and fill with your choice ingredients. Eat the bagels within 1 to 3 days, but you can freeze or refrigerate your bagels if you desire to keep them longer.

Nutrition Facts per Serving:

Total Carbs: 7.2 g

Dietary Fiber: 2.8 g

Net Carbs: 4.4 g

Total Fat: 24.1 g

Protein: 9.2 g

Calories: 273 kcal

MULTI-SEED BAGELS

This fiber-packed bagel recipe does not only taste great, it is great as a 'colon cleanse.' The psyllium fiber provides roughage, and makes your day a bit easier. Moreover, a fiber-packed bagel can keep the doctor away.

Serves: 6

Prep Time: 20 minutes

Cook Time: 55 minutes

Ingredients:

- ¼ cup Psyllium fiber
- 1 cup coconut flour
- 1/3 cup sesame seeds
- ½ cup pumpkin seeds
- ½ cup hemp hearts
- 1 teaspoon sea salt
- 6 egg whites, organic
- 1 tablespoon aluminum-free baking powder

Directions:

1. Preheat oven to 350°F (175°C).
2. In a large bowl, combine the dry ingredients. Mix well.
3. Blend the egg whites in a blender until foamy.
4. Fold in the foamy egg whites to the dry ingredients. Use a spoon to mix them well or use a food processor. The dough should have a crumbly consistency.
5. Add 1 cup boiling water to the dough. Keep on stirring until you form a smoother dough.
6. While the dough may still be crumbly, it will hold its shape when formed into a ball.
7. On a cookie sheet, place one sheet of parchment paper. Make 6 balls from the dough. To form the balls into bagels, make a hole by sticking your thumb through it. Place the formed dough onto the sheet, and use your fingers to press it together, forming a bagel.
8. Sprinkle the bagels with poppy seeds or sesame seeds. For about 55 minutes, bake the bagels at 350°F (175°C). Leave the bagels in the oven after turning off the heat, for a crunchy top.

Nutrition Facts per Serving:

Total Carbs: 28 g

Dietary Fiber: 20 g

Net Carbs: 8 g

Total Fat: 19 g

Protein: 18 g

Calories: 352 kcal

SESAME BUNS

While the recipe is easy to make, there are certain variables that can affect the outcome. Use the lightest and finest coconut flour, and use Psyllium powder that's fine, not flaky. It is also important not to use table salt. Instead, use Celtic sea salt or Himalayan salt.

Serves: 12

Prep Time: 15 minutes

Cook Time: 50 minutes

Ingredients:

- 1 cup coconut flour
- ½ cup pumpkin seeds
- 1 cup sesame seeds (Reserve ½ cup sesame seeds for toppings.)
- 1 cup hot water
- ½ cup Psyllium powder
- 1 tablespoon sea salt
- 8 egg whites
- 1 teaspoon aluminum-free baking powder

Directions:

1. Preheat oven to 350°F (175°C).
2. In a large bowl, combine the dry ingredients. Mix well.
3. Place the eggs whites in a blender and beat until very foamy. Add the whites to the dry ingredients. Use a food processor or a spoon to mix well. The dough should be crumbly.
4. Add 1 cup boiling water and continue to stir until you form a smoother dough. The slightly crumbly dough will keep its shape when formed into a bun.
5. Place ½ cup sesame seeds on a plate. Press the buns into the sesame plate so the seeds stick to the top.
6. On a cookie sheet, place one piece of parchment. Place the sesame buns on the parchment paper.
7. For about 50 minutes, bake the buns at 350°F (175°C).
8. Allow the buns to cool inside the oven to achieve extra-crunchy tops.
9. Remove from oven and serve hot.

Nutrition Facts per Serving:

Total Carbs: 13.5 g

Dietary Fiber: 9.5 g

Net Carbs: 4 g

Total Fat: 6.5 g

Protein: 6.9 g

Calories: 133 kcal

SUGAR-FREE BAGELS

This version of a conventional bagel is guilt-free, and can be eaten with any meal of the day. You can pair it with eggs and bacon for breakfast or a grass-fed steak for lunch. If you desire, you can add a bit of butter on top for a flavorful treat.

Serves: 12

Prep Time: 15 minutes

Cook Time: 25 minutes

Ingredients:

- 1/3 cup sour cream
- 12 eggs
- ¼ cup flaxseed, ground
- ½ teaspoon sea salt
- 1/3 cup coconut flour
- 1 teaspoon baking powder
- 1 cup protein powder

Toppings Ingredients:

- 1 teaspoon oregano, dried

- 1 teaspoon parsley, dried
- ½ teaspoon garlic powder
- 1 teaspoon minced onion, dried
- ½ teaspoon sea salt
- ½ teaspoon basil, dried

Directions:
1. Preheat oven to 350°F (175°C).
2. Place the sour cream and eggs in a stand mixer. Blend until thoroughly combined.
3. In a large bowl, whisk the salt, flaxseed, coconut flour, protein powder, and baking powder together.
4. Gradually pour the dry ingredients into the wet ingredients. Mix until incorporated.
5. Whisk the toppings ingredients together in a small bowl. Set aside.
6. Liberally grease two 6-capacity doughnut pans. Sprinkle approximately 1 teaspoon toppings into each section directly.
7. Evenly pour batter into each section. Sprinkle evenly the remaining seasoning/toppings mixture onto the batter of every bagel.
8. Bake until golden brown or for about 25 minutes.

9. Slightly cool. Remove from pan. Refrigerate the bagels until you are ready to toast and serve them.

Nutrition Facts per Serving:

Total Carbs: 4.2 g

Dietary Fiber: 2.5 g

Net Carbs: 1.7 g

Total Fat: 6.8 g

Protein: 12.1 g

Calories: 134 kcal

Chapter Four: Ketogenic Muffins, Pancakes & Waffles

ALMOND FLOUR WAFFLES

These gluten-free, low-carb waffles are just as tasty as the conventional wheat flour waffles. You can freeze them and reheat them for an easy, quick, and satisfying breakfast.

Serves: 8

Prep Time: 5 minutes

Cook Time: 5 minutes

Ingredients:

- 1 cup sifted almond flour
- ¼ teaspoon salt
- ½ tablespoon baking powder
- 2 tablespoons oil

- 1 cup heavy cream
- 3 eggs

Directions:

1. Whisk together the flour, salt, and baking powder in a large bowl.
2. Stir in the eggs and the oil, and mix until smooth. Gradually add the heavy cream until you achieve the desired batter thickness.
3. Pour the batter into the waffle maker. Cook.
4. Serve hot and plain or topped with grass-fed butter.

Nutrition Facts per Serving:

Total Carbs: 3 g

Dietary Fiber: 2 g

Net Carbs: 1 g

Total Fat: 24 g

Protein: 6 g

Calories: 245 kcal

CHEESE MUFFINS

The Ketogenic Diet does not deprive you of everything. You can still eat cheese and dairy, in moderation. This recipe can satisfy your cheese cravings, and you can enjoy the muffins for breakfast or a mid-morning snack. You can even consume the muffins as a lunch or dinner side dish.

Serves: 12

Prep Time: 15 minutes

Cook Time: 25 minutes

Ingredients:

- 2 cups almond flour
- ¼ teaspoon salt
- ½ teaspoon baking soda
- 2 eggs
- ½ teaspoon thyme, dried
- 1/8 cup butter, melted
- 1 cup sour cream
- ½ cup muenster, shredded
- 1 cup Colby jack or cheddar, shredded

Directions:

1. Preheat oven to 400°F (205°C). Place cupcake papers inside the muffin holes of a standard 12-count muffin tin.
2. In a bowl, whisk together the dry ingredients and almond flour. In another bowl, lightly beat the eggs. Mix in the butter and sour cream.
3. Fold in the liquid mixture to the dry ingredients mixture. If you find the batter too thick, add one tablespoon of heavy cream or water.
4. Add the cheese and stir until the cheese is distributed evenly.
5. Spoon the batter into the muffin cups, and fill each up ¾ full.
6. For 5 minutes, bake at 400°F (205°C). Turn down the temperature to 350°F (175°C), and bake for a further 20 minutes or until the muffins achieve a golden color.
7. Allow to cool slightly. Serve hot with butter.

Nutrition Facts per Serving:

Total Carbs: 5 g

Dietary Fiber: 3 g

Net Carbs: 2 g

Total Fat: 15 g

Protein: 6 g

Calories: 166 kcal

CREAM CHEESE PANCAKES

These cheesy pancakes are extremely filling, and are so easy to make. Serve them with grass-fed butter and maple syrup, and you end up with pancakes that taste similar to French toast – only without the guilt.

Serves: 1

Prep Time: 5 minutes

Cook Time: 10 minutes

Ingredients:

- 2 eggs
- 2 ounces cream cheese
- 1 tablespoon coconut flour
- ½ teaspoon cinnamon
- ½ to 1 packet stevia

Directions:

1. Beat or blend together the ingredients until the batter is smooth and free of lumps.

2. Two pancakes is equivalent to one serving. On medium-high, heat up a non-stick skillet or pan with coconut oil or salted butter.
3. Ladle the batter on to the pan. Heat until bubbles begin to form on top. Flip over, and cook until the other side is sufficiently browned.
4. Serve. Top with sugar-free maple syrup and grass-fed butter.

Nutrition Facts per Serving:

Total Carbs: 8 g

Dietary Fiber: 3 g

Net Carbs: 5 g

Total Fat: 29 g

Protein: 17 g

Calories: 365 kcal

GLUTEN-FREE LOW-CARB PANCAKES

These gluten-free pancakes can be consumed by people following the Paleo diet. These pancakes with coconut flour and almond flour, which are easy to make, are fluffy and delicious. You will be wanting these pancakes for many mornings to come.

Serves: 11

Prep Time: 5 minutes

Cook Time: 15 minutes

Ingredients:

- ¼ cup coconut flour
- 1 cup almond flour
- 1 teaspoon baking powder, gluten-free
- 6 large eggs
- 2 tablespoons Erythritol (or any choice sweetener)
- ¼ cup almond milk (or any choice milk), unsweetened

Directions:

1. In a bowl, whisk all ingredients until smooth and free of lumps.

2. On the stovetop, over medium-low to medium heat, preheat an oiled pan. Ladle the batter on to the hot pan. Form the batter into circles.
3. Cover the pan and cook for 1 ½ to 2 minutes, until bubbles begin to form at the top.
4. Flip the pancakes over and cook for another 1 ½ to 2 minutes, or until the other side is golden brown.
5. Repeat the procedure with the remaining batter.
6. Serve hot with honey and grass-fed butter.

Nutrition Facts per Serving:

Total Carbs: 4 g

Dietary Fiber: 3 g

Net Carbs: 1 g

Total Fat: 8 g

Protein: 6 g

Calories: 107 kcal

LEMON BLUEBERRY MUFFINS

You would love these muffins on a chilly morning. Spread some warm grass-fed butter on each muffin, and you got yourself a deliciously low-carb breakfast. As compared to conventional muffins, these low-carb muffins are more filling and richer tasting.

Serves: 15

Prep Time: 15 minutes

Cook Time: 20 minutes

Ingredients:

- 1 cup heavy cream
- 2 cups almond flour
- 1/8 cup butter, melted
- 2 eggs
- ½ teaspoon baking soda
- 5 packets artificial sweetener like stevia or Splenda
- ½ teaspoon lemon zest, dried
- ½ teaspoon lemon flavoring or extract
- 4 ounces blueberries, fresh
- ¼ teaspoon salt

Directions:

1. Preheat the oven to 350°F (175°C). Put cupcake papers in the muffin holes.
2. In a bowl, mix the cream and almond flour. One at a time, add the eggs. Stir the mixture until well mixed.
3. To the mixture, add sweetener, butter, baking soda, spices, and flavoring. Fold in the blueberries and stir until distributed evenly.
4. Spoon the mixture into the muffin pan. Fill each cupcake paper to about ½ full. Bake the muffins until golden or for about 20 minutes.
5. Allow to slightly cool. Serve hot with butter.

Nutrition Facts per Serving:

Total Carbs: 6 g

Dietary Fiber: 2 g

Net Carbs: 4 g

Total Fat: 17 g

Protein: 5 g

Calories: 184 kcal

LOW-CARB CINNAMON WAFFLES

If you love cinnamon rolls, this recipe could be a hit with you, and may bring back memories of your childhood. This version, however, is far healthier than the conventional cinnamon rolls. The waffle is packed with protein and healthy fat to keep you going.

Serves: 1

Prep Time: 5 minutes

Cook Time: 5 minutes

Ingredients:

- 6 tablespoons almond flour
- 1 tablespoon Erythritol
- 2 eggs, large
- ½ teaspoon cinnamon
- ¼ teaspoon baking soda
- ½ teaspoon vanilla extract
- Non-stick spray

Cream Cheese Frosting Ingredients:

- 1 tablespoon Erythritol

- 2 tablespoons cream cheese
- 1 tablespoon heavy cream
- ¼ teaspoon vanilla extract
- 2 teaspoons leftover batter
- ¼ teaspoon cinnamon

Directions:

1. In a bowl, mix all the dry ingredients together. Add the wet ingredients to the dry ingredients. Mix well until smooth and free of lumps.
2. Pour the batter into the waffle iron. Meanwhile, mix together the cream cheese filling ingredients.
3. Slice the waffle into quarters. Evenly spread the cream cheese over half of the waffle.
4. Place the waffle quarters (non-frosted) on top to make a waffle sandwich.
5. You can eat the waffle as an entire meal. You can also consume half the waffle as a snack.

Nutrition Facts per Serving:

Total Carbs: 13 g

Dietary Fiber: 6 g

Net Carbs: 7 g

Total Fat: 50 g

Protein: 22.8 g

Calories: 542 kcal

LOW-CARB SOUR CREAM BLUEBERRY MUFFINS

This protein-packed breakfast food item can satisfy you throughout the morning. Add a bit of grass-fed butter on top, and pair it with your favorite fruit. You can enjoy this muffin with bacon or eggs. These muffins are a perfect way to power up your day.

Serves: 15

Prep Time: 15 minutes

Cook Time: 20 minutes

Ingredients:

- 2 cups almond flour
- ½ teaspoon baking soda
- ¼ cup Erythritol
- 1 cup sour cream
- ½ teaspoon salt
- 2 eggs
- 4 ounces blueberries, fresh
- 1/8 cup butter, melted

Directions:

1. Preheat the oven to 350°F (175°C). Place cupcake papers inside the individual muffin holes of your muffin tin.
2. In a large bowl, whisk together the dry ingredients and the almond flour.
3. In another bowl, beat the eggs lightly. Add in the butter and sour cream. Mix until thoroughly combined.
4. Combine the almond flour mixture with the sour cream mixture. Stir until thoroughly mixed. Add the blueberries until they are evenly incorporated.
5. Spoon the batter into the muffin cups, and fill each muffin paper up to ½ full.
6. Bake the muffins until golden or for about 20 minutes.
7. Allow to slightly cool. Serve hot with butter.

Nutrition Facts per Serving:

Total Carbs: 5 g

Dietary Fiber: 2 g

Net Carbs: 3 g

Total Fat: 13 g

Protein: 5 g

Calories: 147 kcal

Chapter Five: Ketogenic Pizza Crust

CAULIFLOWER CRUST

When you are trying to eat healthy, you do not have to deny yourself the occasional treat. If you want to eat guilt-free pizza, this recipe offers you an excellent alternative. This cauliflower-based crust lets you enjoy your favorite pizza while letting you stick to your Ketogenic diet lifestyle.

Serves: 1 pizza crust

Prep Time: 20 minutes

Cook Time: 30 minutes

Ingredients:

- 1 piece cauliflower head, stalk removed
- ¼ cup Parmesan, grated
- ½ cup mozzarella, shredded
- ½ teaspoon kosher salt
- ½ teaspoon oregano, dried

- ¼ teaspoon garlic powder
- 2 eggs, beaten lightly

Directions:

1. Preheat oven to 400°F (205°C). Use parchment paper to line a baking sheet.
2. Cut the cauliflower head into florets. In a food processor, pulse the cauliflower until fine.
3. Place the cauliflower in a steamer basket. Steam it and drain well. Allow to cool.
4. In a bowl, mix the fine cauliflower together with the Parmesan, mozzarella, salt, oregano, eggs, and garlic powder.
5. Place the mixture in the center of the lined baking sheet and form into a circle to look like a pizza crust.
6. Bake for about 20 minutes.
7. Add your toppings of choice and bake for another 10 minutes.
8. Serve hot. Enjoy.

Nutrition Facts per Serving:

Total Carbs: 26.1 g

Dietary Fiber: 6.6 g

Net Carbs: 19.5 g

Total Fat: 21.05 g

Protein: 49.11 g

Calories: 483 kcal

EASY ALMOND FLOUR PIZZA CRUST

This pizza crust recipe is not only ketogenic, it is dairy-free, gluten-free, and Paleo-and vegan-friendly, too. Moreover, with only four ingredients to make, this is one of the easiest keto dough recipes that you can use as a base for your favorite pizza toppings.

Serves: 8

Prep Time: 5 minutes

Cook Time: 15 minutes

Ingredients:

- 2 cups almond flour
- 2 eggs, large
- 2 tablespoons coconut oil, melted
- ½ teaspoon sea salt

Directions:

1. Use parchment paper to line a baking sheet. Preheat oven to 350°F (175°C).
2. In a bowl, mix the ingredients together until you form a dough. You can manually mix it or use a food processor.

3. Form the dough into a ball. Put in between two parchment paper sheets, and roll out the dough to ¼" thick.

4. Remove the parchment paper piece on top. Place the crust on a pizza pan. Use a toothpick to poke the crust a few times to prevent bubbling.

5. Bake until golden or for 15 to 20 minutes.

6. When you want to use the crust to make pizza, top with you preferred toppings. Return to the oven until edges are crispy and cheese is bubbling or for 10 to 15 minutes.

7. If you are sensitive to coconut oil's flavor, you can use ghee or butter.

Nutrition Facts per Serving:

Total Carbs: 6 g

Dietary Fiber: 3 g

Net Carbs: 3 g

Total Fat: 19 g

Protein: 8 g

Calories: 211 kcal

LOW-CARB PIZZA CRUST

Since the base of the crust is cauliflower, you cannot expect a crispy and thin pizza crust. You may have to use a fork to eat this pizza crust. One thing is for sure, though. This crust recipe is delicious, low-carb, and completely satisfying.

Serves: 8

Prep Time: 20 minutes

Cook Time: 20 minutes

Ingredients:

- 1 tablespoon olive oil
- 1 ½ ounces white onion, minced
- 1 piece cauliflower head, organic (Trim and chop it into small pieces.)
- ¼ cup water
- 2 tablespoons butter
- 3 eggs
- 2 cups mozzarella cheese, shredded (In the food processor, chop the cheese into smaller bits.)
- 2 teaspoons Italian seasoning

- 1 teaspoon fennel seed
- ¼ cup Parmesan cheese, grated

Directions:

1. Grease a 17"x11" cookie sheet with olive oil. Preheat the oven to 450°F (230°C).
2. In a large lidded skillet, melt the butter. Add the cauliflower and onion. Over low to medium heat, sauté the vegetables until the cauliflower is nearly done.
3. Add the water. Cover the skillet with its lid, and steam until the cauliflower is softened completely. Remove from heat. Set it aside and allow to cool.
4. Once cooled, measure out three cups of the cauliflower and put it in a food processor. Blend it to a smooth consistency. Into a mixing bowl, scrape the pureed cauliflower.
5. Add the mozzarella cheese, eggs, parmesan, and spices into the cauliflower mixture. Combine the ingredients thoroughly.
6. Use a spatula to spread the dough on the cookie sheet. Make sure your spread dough is even.
7. Bake the dough at 450°F (230°C) for around 20 minutes, or until the edges are browned and the surface looks cooked.
8. Remove from oven. Add pizza sauce on it, and then add your desired toppings. You may add vegetables, pepperoni, and cheese. Put the pizza back in the oven and bake until the cheese melts or for around 5 minutes.

Nutrition Facts per Serving:

Total Carbs: 5.18 g

Dietary Fiber: 1.49 g

Net Carbs: 3.69 g

Total Fat: 9.49 g

Protein: 14.05 g

Calories: 161.13 kcal

KETO CAULIFLOWER CRUST

Cauliflower can be a substitute for the standard wheat flour-based pizza crust. You can enjoy your pizza, and you can still control your weight. The cheese adds maximum flavor to this already-tasty crust.

Serves: 4

Prep Time: 20 minutes

Cook Time: 30 to 35 minutes

Ingredients:

- 1 egg (large), beaten slightly
- 1 pound cauliflower
- 1 teaspoon oregano, dried
- 1 cup mozzarella cheese
- 4 ounces black olives
- 1 cup feta cheese
- White onion
- A pinch of black pepper
- ½ cup tomato puree
- A pinch of salt

Directions:

1. Chop the cauliflower head into florets. Place the florets in a food process or blender. Pulse until you achieve a rice-like consistency. Alternatively, you may use a cheese grater to process the cauliflower.

2. In a pot, boil water. Add the cauliflower rice and boil for about 5 minutes. Drain off the water. Cool the cauliflower rice for a few minutes.

3. Place the cauliflower into a cheesecloth and fold the cloth around the cauliflower. Squeeze the cloth as hard as possible.

4. Place the already-dry cauliflower into a large bowl. Add the salt, oregano, egg, and pepper. Mix well. You may want to use your hands for this.

5. Use parchment paper to line a baking sheet. Spread out the cauliflower mixture into the pizza crust shape you desire.

6. The dough should be about 1/3 inch thick, with the edges a bit higher for that pizza crust effect.

7. Place the dough in an oven preheated to 400°F (205°C) and bake for around 30 to 35 minutes, or until the crust has a golden brown color.

8. Remove the crust from the oven and pour the tomato puree. Add the mozzarella, some onion, crumbled feta cheese, and black olives. Pop it back in the oven and bake for 5 to 10 minutes more, or until the cheese is bubbling.

9. Remove from oven, and slightly cool. Serve and enjoy.

Nutrition Facts per Serving:

Total Carbs: 9.5 g

Dietary Fiber: 3.5 g

Net Carbs: 6 g

Total Fat: 17.5 g

Protein: 17 g

Calories: 262.5 kcal

PARMESAN AND ALMOND PIZZA CRUST

The almond flour in the crust recipe is a perfect replacement for conventional wheat flour. Pair it with parmesan, and you get a crust with a nutty and cheesy flavor that complements well with any toppings that you add.

Serves: 8

Prep Time: 10 minutes

Cook Time: 20 to 25 minutes

Ingredients:

- 1 whole egg, large
- 1 tablespoon olive oil, extra virgin
- ¼ cup water, from the tap
- ½ cup Parmesan cheese, grated
- 1 ½ cups almond flour, blanched
- ½ teaspoon xylitol
- ½ teaspoon baking powder
- ¾ teaspoon oregano
- ¾ teaspoon dried basil
- ¼ teaspoon red pepper flakes, crushed

Directions:

1. Whisk the wet ingredients (water, egg, and oil) together in a bowl. Set aside.
2. Mix together the remainder of the dry ingredients. Stir to blend thoroughly. While spices are optional, they add flavor to the dough. You may add up to ¼ teaspoon chili flakes and ½ teaspoon garlic powder.
3. Add the wet ingredients to the dry ingredients. Stir thoroughly so you can form a thick dough.
4. Grease 2 parchment paper sheets, and roll the dough between the parchments. Shape the dough into a square or thin circle to fit a baking sheet or pizza pan.
5. Bake the dough at 375°C (190°C) for 20 to 25 minutes, or until crisp and golden at the edges.
6. Let cool inside oven for about 20 minutes to form a crispy crust.
7. Top the crust with your desired toppings, and place the crust back in the broiler or oven for several minutes to cook the toppings.
8. Serve hot. Enjoy.

Nutrition Facts per Serving:

Total Carbs: 3.75 g

Dietary Fiber: 2.6 g

Net Carbs: 1.15 g

Total Fat: 14.3 g

Protein: 7.2 g

Calories: 167 kcal

Chapter Six: Ketogenic Crackers

CHEESY KETO CRACKERS

These cheesy crackers are perfect for the holiday season as well as for parties. Your gatherings can have that healthy twist, and these crackers are excellent for nibbling.

Serves: 8

Prep Time: 20 minutes

Cook Time: 40 minutes

Ingredients:

- ½ cup flaxseed meal
- 1 cup almond flour
- 1 cup parmesan cheese, grated
- 2 tablespoons Psyllium husks, whole
- ¼ teaspoon black pepper
- 1 teaspoon sea salt or Himalayan salt

- 1 cup water

Directions:

1. Mix together the flaxseed meal, almond flour, Psyllium, pepper, and salt. Add the grated parmesan into the almond flour mix, and mix thoroughly.

2. Add the water. Use a spatula or your hands to mix well. Allow the dough to sit for 10 to 15 minutes.

3. Preheat the oven to 325°F (165°C).

4. Halve the dough equally. Place one dough half on a parchment paper. Place another parchment paper sheet on top. Roll out until the dough is 1/8 inch (1/4 cm) thick.

5. To get a rectangular shape, use the parchment paper's edges to fold over the dough from the sides. Using the rolling pin, roll once more to flatten out. Repeat when necessary.

6. Cut dough into 16 equal parts using a pizza cutter. Repeat the procedure for the other half of the dough.

7. Put the prepared sheet dough in the oven and bake for 40 to 45 minutes. You can pair the crackers with salmon pate, cheesy bacon dip, marinara sauce, or guacamole.

8. You can store the crackers for 5 days at room temperature, or up to 3 months in the freezer.

Nutrition Facts per Serving:

Total Carbs: 6.3 g

Dietary Fiber: 4.5 g

Net Carbs: 1.7 g

Total Fat: 13.4 g

Protein: 8.4 g

Calories: 168 kcal

GRAIN-FREE KETO CRACKERS

This recipe is simple to prepare, and you only need a handful of ingredients. You only need to make sure that you properly prepare your chia seeds. These versatile, nutty crackers can be paired with smoked salmon, avocado, or cream cheese. You can even pair them with prosciutto.

Serves: 8

Prep Time: 10 minutes

Cook Time: 45 minutes

Ingredients:

- 4 tablespoons hemp hearts
- 4 tablespoons chia seeds
- 2 tablespoons olive oil, extra virgin
- ½ cup almond flour
- A pinch of sea salt
- ½ cup water (to soak the seeds)

Directions:

1. Soak the chia seeds for an hour in water, and preheat the oven to 200°F (95°C).
2. After half an hour, the chia seeds should be gelatinous and absorb the water. Their consistency should be thick when stirred. If picked up with a spoon, the seeds should stick to the spoon.
3. If the seeds are still runny and wet, add another tablespoon of chia seeds. Wait for a further 10 minutes.
4. Add the rest of the ingredients to the chia seeds, and mix thoroughly to form a dough. You should be able to form a ball with this.
5. Place the dough on a parchment paper sheet. Cover the dough ball with cling wrap plastic. Roll it out using a rolling pin or a wine bottle.
6. Roll the dough as thin as possible, as thin as ¼". Gently peel off the plastic sheet.
7. Place the parchment paper over a cookie sheet. Make sure not to break the rolled dough. For about 45 minutes or until the dough is slightly browned and dried, bake at 200°F (95°C).
8. Allow to cool, and cut the sheet into 2" cracker squares with a knife. Peel the crackers from the bottom parchment paper. Keep in an airtight container.

Nutrition Facts per Serving:

Total Carbs: 4.25 g

Dietary Fiber: 3.25 g

Net Carbs: 1 g

Total Fat: 10.3 g

Protein: 3.75 g

Calories: 122 kcal

KETO PESTO CRACKERS

These crackers combine everybody's favorite Italian taste with a buttery crisp texture. The flavor is a wonderful combination of basil, black pepper, and garlic, with a whiff of cayenne to awaken your taste buds.

Serves: 6

Prep Time: 15 minutes

Cook Time: 17 minutes

Ingredients:

- 1 ¼ cups almond flour
- ½ teaspoon salt
- ¼ teaspoon black pepper, ground
- ¼ teaspoon basil, dried
- ½ teaspoon baking powder
- 1 clove pressed garlic
- A pinch of cayenne pepper
- 3 tablespoons butter
- 2 tablespoons basil pesto

Directions:

1. Use parchment paper to line a cookie tray. Preheat the oven to 325°F (165°C).

2. In a bowl, combine pepper, almond flour, baking powder, and salt. Whisk the dry ingredients together until smooth. Add the garlic, cayenne, and basil, and stir until combined evenly.

3. Add the basil pesto. Whisk until you achieve a dough with coarse crumbs.

4. Use a fork or your fingers to cut the butter into the mixture. Continue with the procedure until can form the dough into a ball.

5. Place the dough on the prepared cookie tray. Spread the dough out into a thickness of 1 ½ mm. Make sure the thickness is consistent so the crackers evenly bake.

6. Place the pan in the oven and bake until you achieve a golden brown color or for 14 to 17 minutes.

7. Remove from the oven, and cut the crackers into your preferred shape and size. You may also let the cracker sheet cool down, and then break them into pieces.

Nutrition Facts per Serving:

Total Carbs: 5.5 g

Dietary Fiber: 2.5 g

Net Carbs: 3 g

Total Fat: 19.83 g

Protein: 5.3 g

Calories: 209.83 kcal

LOW-CARB FLAXSEED CRACKERS

Because of these crackers' plain flavor, they can be perfectly paired with salty food items like cured meats, dips, and cheese. With these crackers' crispy texture, you may find it hard to limit yourself with just one serving.

Serves: 13

Prep Time: 10 minutes

Cook Time: 10 minutes

Ingredients:

- ¼ cup flaxseed
- ¾ cup flaxseed meal
- 1 egg
- 1/3 cup parmesan cheese, grated finely
- ½ cup water

Directions:

1. Preheat the oven to 390°F (200°C).
2. In a medium bowl, combine the flaxseed, flaxseed meal, and parmesan. Mix thoroughly.

3. Add the egg and water. Vigorously stir until you can form a dough. Make sure to thoroughly combine the dry ingredients.
4. Tear off dough balls the size of teaspoons. Put them on a parchment-lined baking tray. Cover the balls with a sheet of parchment paper and use a flat object to flatten out the dough to a thinness of 2mm. A measuring cup or a glass bottom can do the trick.
5. For 8 minutes, bake the crackers. Turn the crackers over and bake for 2 more minutes. Depending on your baking trays and oven size, you may need to cook your crackers in batches.
6. After the crackers have finished baking, turn off the oven. Crisp the crackers for 20 more minutes.

Nutrition Facts per Serving:

Total Carbs: 6 g

Dietary Fiber: 6 g

Net Carbs: N/A

Total Fat: 7 g

Protein: 6 g

Calories: 110 kcal

LOW-CARB SEA SALT CRACKERS

These crackers are crunchy, salty, and crispy. They can be paired with cheese and dips. They also go well with antipasto plates. Just make sure you thoroughly bake and dry out these crackers, as under-cooked crackers can rapidly become stale.

Serves: 7

Prep Time: 15 minutes

Cook Time: 12 minutes

Ingredients:

- ¼ cup sesame seeds
- ¾ cup flaxseed meal
- 1/3 cup parmesan cheese, grated finely
- ½ cup water
- 1 egg
- 1 tablespoon sea salt

Directions:

1. Preheat the oven to 375°F (190°C). In a medium bowl, combine the flaxseed meal, parmesan cheese, and sesame seeds. Mix the ingredients thoroughly.

2. Add the egg and water. Stir vigorously until you can form a firm dough.

3. Tear off dough balls the size of teaspoons. Place them on a lined baking sheet. Cover with a small parchment paper square. Use a flat object to flatten out the dough to a thickness of 2 mm. You can use a flat-bottomed water glass for this.

4. Onto each cracker, sprinkle a few sea salt flakes. Gently press down to make sure the salt flakes stick.

5. Bake the keto crackers for 8 minutes. Flip them over and bake for 3 minutes more. Depending on the size of your oven trays or ovens, you may have to do batch cooking.

6. After you are done baking, turn off the oven. Allow the crackers to completely crisp and dry out.

7. Remove from oven and cool off the crackers completely. Store in an airtight, dry jar.

Nutrition Facts per Serving:

Total Carbs: 10 g

Dietary Fiber: 9 g

Net Carbs: 1 g

Total Fat: 12 g

Protein: 11 g

Calories: 194 kcal

Chapter Seven: Ketogenic Breadsticks

CAULIFLOWER CHEESE BREADSTICKS

This recipe is low-carb, gluten-free, keto-friendly, and cheesy. You can also freeze the cauliflower crust and just thaw it when you need it.

Serves: 8

Prep Time: 10 minutes

Cook Time: 40 minutes

Ingredients:

- 1 piece cauliflower head, large (This can make 4 cups of riced cauliflower.)
- 2 cups mozzarella
- 4 eggs
- 4 cloves garlic, minced
- 3 teaspoons oregano
- Pepper and salt to taste

- 1 cup mozzarella cheese for topping

Directions:

1. Prepare one large baking dish or 2 pizza dishes lined with parchment paper.
2. Preheat the oven to 425°F (220°C).
3. Chop up the cauliflower into florets. Place them in a food processor, and pulse until the cauliflower looks like rice.
4. Put the cauliflower in a microwave-safe container. Cover the lid, and microwave for 10 minutes. Release the steam and allow the cauliflower to cool.
5. In a large bowl, combine the cauliflower with the eggs, 2 cups mozzarella, garlic, oregano, salt, and pepper. Mix until thoroughly combined.
6. Divide the dough and put each half on to the prepared baking sheet.
7. Without the toppings, bake the crust for around 25 minutes or until golden and nice. After 25 or so minutes, sprinkle the rest of the mozzarella cheese.
8. Place the cauliflower crust back in the oven for 5 minutes more or until the mozzarella has melted. Slice into sticks. Serve and enjoy.

Nutrition Facts per Serving:

Total Carbs: 3.36 g

Dietary Fiber: 0.9 g

Net Carbs: 2.46 g

Total Fat: 13.32 g

Protein: 13.22 g

Calories: 185 kcal

CHEESY GARLIC BREADSTICKS

Mozzarella cheese is an excellent base for low-carbohydrate breads like pie crust, pizza dough, and breadsticks. The cheese compensates for the lack of gluten in such gluten-free breads.

Serves: 6

Prep Time: 10 minutes

Cook Time: 15 minutes

Ingredients:

- 1 cup almond flour (Provide extra for kneading.)
- 2 tablespoons coconut flour
- 3 tablespoons whey protein powder, unflavored
- 2 teaspoons baking powder
- ½ teaspoon salt
- ½ teaspoon garlic powder
- 1 ½ cups mozzarella cheese, grated
- ¼ cup butter, melted
- 2 large eggs
- ½ teaspoon xanthan gum, optional

Toppings Ingredients:

- 2 tablespoons parmesan, grated
- 3 tablespoons butter, softened
- ½ teaspoon garlic powder

Directions:

1. Preheat the oven to 400°F (205°C).
2. In a bowl, whisk the whey protein, almond flour, baking powder, coconut flour, salt, garlic powder, and xanthan gum. In another bowl, place the mozzarella cheese. Melt it in the microwave.
3. Stir the butter, eggs, and dry mix into the mozzarella cheese until you form a dough. If the cheese starts to harden, microwave the ball of dough for 5 to 10 seconds to incorporate all the ingredients in the dough. More almond flour may be needed if you find the dough too sticky.
4. Put the dough ball between two large parchment paper sheets. Use a rolling pin to roll the dough out into a circle with a thickness of ¼" inch.
5. Peel off the top parchment paper piece, and place the dough on a baking sheet. Use a knife of pizza cutter to cut the dough into stick-like pieces.

6. Mix the toppings ingredients and spread them all over the dough. Bake until the top starts to brown or for 10 to 15 minutes.
7. Remove to slightly cool. Serve warm and enjoy.

Nutrition Facts per Serving:

Total Carbs: 9.6 g

Dietary Fiber: 3.8 g

Net Carbs: 5.8 g

Total Fat: 33.8 g

Protein: 24 g

Calories: 425 kcal

KETO BREADSTICKS

Yes, you can make breadsticks out of cauliflower. These keto breadsticks are infused with garlic, fresh herbs, and cheese atop a cauliflower crust. The breadsticks taste just like cheesy bread.

Serves: 5

Prep Time: 15 minutes

Cook Time: 15 minutes

Ingredients:

- 1 piece raw cauliflower head, riced
- ½ cup parmesan cheese, shaved
- ½ cup mozzarella cheese, shredded
- 1 large egg
- ½ tablespoon basil, freshly chopped
- ½ tablespoon garlic, freshly minced
- ½ tablespoon Italian flat-leaf pastry, freshly chopped
- 1 teaspoon salt
- ¾ cup mozzarella cheese, shredded
- ½ teaspoon black pepper, ground

Directions:

1. Preheat the oven to 425°F (220°C). Use parchment paper or a silicon baking mat to line a baking tray.
2. Rice the cauliflower by first breaking it down into florets. Place it in a food processor, and pulse it until you achieve a rice-like texture.
3. In a bowl, mix ½ shredded mozzarella, the riced cauliflower, ½ cup parmesan, 1 egg, ½ tablespoon basil, ½ tablespoon garlic, ½ tablespoon parsley, ½ teaspoon black pepper, and ½ teaspoon salt until combined thoroughly and the mixture holds together.
4. Put the mixture on the lined baking tray. Spread out into a 1/4" thick x 9" long x 7" wide rectangle.
5. For 10 to 12 minutes, bake the cauliflower crust in the preheated oven. Remove from oven. Top with the ¾ cup mozzarella. Return to the oven to continue baking and until the cheese is beginning to brown.
6. For about 10 minutes, cool the crust and cut it into breadsticks.
7. Garnish with parmesan and fresh herbs. Serve and enjoy.

Nutrition Facts per Serving:

Total Carbs: 7 g

Dietary Fiber: 2 g

Net Carbs: 5 g

Total Fat: 4.5 g

Protein: 8 g

Calories: 100 kcal

PIZZA BREADSTICKS

These breadsticks are cheesy and crispy, and you do not have to deprive yourself of this pizza-like treat. You can serve these breadsticks with low-carb ranch dressing or tomato sauce.

Serves: 4

Prep Time: 20 minutes

Cook Time: 15 minutes

Ingredients:

- 1 cup and 2 tablespoons mozzarella cheese, shredded (part-skim, low-moisture)
- 3 tablespoons coconut flour
- 6 tablespoons almond flour
- ½ teaspoon baking powder
- 1 egg, beaten
- 4 tablespoons butter
- ¼ teaspoon salt
- ¼ teaspoon oregano
- 1/8 teaspoon pepper, freshly ground
- ¼ teaspoon garlic powder

- ½ teaspoon dried parsley
- ¼ teaspoon red pepper flakes
- 1 clove garlic
- 1 cup shredded cheddar cheese
- ½ cup shredded pepper jack cheese
- 1 tablespoon olive oil, extra virgin

Directions:

1. Preheat the oven to 400°F (205°C).
2. In a microwave, melt the mozzarella cheese for 25 seconds or until it forms a melted cheese ball. In a large bowl, combine coconut flour, almond flour, 2 tablespoons butter, baking powder, garlic powder, egg, pepper, salt, and parsley.
3. Put the wet dough mix on a chopping board. Mix together with the mozzarella and knead to integrate the cheese into the flour mix. Keep on kneading as it takes about 3 to 4 minutes to get a proper consistency.
4. On a baking sheet, place a sheet of parchment paper. Roll out the dough into a circular form, and put it on the baking sheet. Use olive oil to drizzle the dough. For 8 minutes, bake the dough or until the edges become crispy and golden brown.
5. In a microwave-safe bowl, combine the garlic clove and 2 tablespoons butter. For 45 seconds, microwave until the melted butter is garlic-infused. Rub this evenly on the crust.

6. Top the buttered crust with oregano, red pepper, flakes, and the cheddar and pepper jack cheeses.
7. Bake for 7 minutes more, or until the cheese is bubbly and melted.
8. Slice into sticks. Serve and enjoy.

Nutrition Facts per Serving:

Total Carbs: 9.6 g

Dietary Fiber: 3.1 g

Net Carbs: 6.5 g

Total Fat: 37 g

Protein: 19.7 g

Calories: 495 kcal

SESAME LOW-CARB BREADSTICKS

Lupin is not your average flour for a ketogenic dish. However, they are the best for keto baking and cooking. Lupins are legumes that are similar to peanuts. If you are sensitive to peanuts, chances are, you may also be sensitive to lupins. If so, it is best to use alternative flours like almond or coconut.

Serves: 5

Prep Time: 5 minutes

Cook Time: 20 minutes

Ingredients:

- 1 egg white, derived from 1 medium egg
- ½ teaspoon sesame seeds
- 1 teaspoon Himalayan pink salt, fine
- 30 grams lupin flour
- 1 tablespoon olive oil, extra virgin

Directions:

1. Whisk the egg white lightly. Add ½ tablespoon olive oil, ½ teaspoon salt, and lupin flour.

2. Mix thoroughly the ingredients. Afterwards, hand knead the dough until it is not too sticky but still soft. Depending on the weight of the egg white, you may need to a bit of water or more lupin flour.

3. Preheat the oven to 320°F (160°C).

4. Place a sheet of parchment paper on an oven tray. Smear the sesame seeds, ½ teaspoon salt, and ½ tablespoon olive oil on it.

5. Divide the dough into five parts. Roll each part while stretching over a hard surface. Shape them into breadsticks.

6. Place the breadsticks on the parchment paper and roll them so they get evenly coated with the sesame seeds, oil, and salt.

7. Bake for 25 minutes. Turn off the oven. Slightly open the oven door and allow the breadsticks to dry up further.

8. Once cooled, remove from the oven. Enjoy. Each breadstick has a 1-centimeter diameter and has a length of 15 to 17 centimeters.

9. The breadsticks can be kept for a few days in a plastic sealed container. However, they can become stale. If this happens, all you have to do is reheat the breadsticks for a few minutes, and they will become crunchy again.

Nutrition Facts per Serving:

Total Carbs: 5.16 g

Dietary Fiber: 1.16 g

Net Carbs: 4 g

Total Fat: 17.13 g

Protein: 13.88 g

Calories: 246 kcal

Conclusion

With your doubts regarding cooking on the ketogenic diet diminishing, you can confidently whip up those sumptuous breads that you can eat for breakfast, lunch, dinner, and snacks. You can substitute some ingredients as long as they are still related. You can experiment and use coconut flour in place of almond flour. You can add chocolate to your favorite pancake recipe. It is all up to you.

What is great with this book is that it shows that you can never deprive yourself of your favorite food while you are on the keto diet. You can still consume healthier versions of bread, pizza, crackers, pancakes, waffles, muffins, and many other baked and flour-based goods.

Baking bread and other related products is just part of the broad spectrum that comprises the Ketogenic diet. As you discover that you can easily make your favorite baked goods, in time, you will branch out to make other dishes that can be categorized as keto-friendly. Soon, you will pair your breads with protein-rich and fat-rich dishes like organic steaks, pork, and poultry.

As you ease into the ketogenic diet beginning with these 35 recipes, you will reap the benefits of the diet in no time. The ketogenic diet can be a long-term solution to achieve optimal health. Despite the high amount of healthy fat you consume in the diet, you may find out that you are losing a healthy amount of weight. With such weight loss, you can attain mental clarity, be free from suffering from medical conditions, and live a happy and meaningful life with your smart food choices.

Author's Note

Thank you so much for taking the time to read my book. I hope you have enjoyed reading this book as much as I've enjoyed writing it. If you enjoyed this book, please consider leaving a review on Amazon. Your support really means a lot and keeps me going.

If you have any questions, please don't hesitate to contact me at ask@cleaneatingspirit.com

Don't forget to follow me on Facebook and Instagram for more information related to health and wellness.

Facebook: https://www.facebook.com/cleaneatingspirit

Instagram: https://www.instagram.com/cleaneatingspirit